Gluten Free Fitness Bundle

The Ultimate Beginners Guide To A Gluten Free Diet

Beginners Guide to 10 Tasty Diet Meals to Lose Weight

&

The Ultimate Guide to Becoming a Label Reading Master

By Scott Jay Marshall II

©2016

Disclaimer

The books in this bundle were written as a simple guide to beginning a gluten free diet in regards to simple meals as well as beginning to read labels. This does not replace any medical advice received from a medical professional nor is this book providing any medical advice. If you ever have a severe reaction to a food item you have consumed, immediately schedule an appointment with your doctor to address the issue. The writer, distributors, and all others involved with this book are not responsible for any negative results that manifest from following the suggestions in this work. Always practice the utmost diligence when eating new foods if you have a food allergy or autoimmune disease.

Introduction To The Bundle

Welcome to the bundle!

After the success that "Beginners Guide To 10 Tasty Diet Meals To Lose Weight" and "Ultimate Guide To Becoming A Label Reading Master" generated and the masses of people that benefited from the two books I decided that it would be a smart next move to put the two together in a bundle. This would make it much easier for a health and fitness minded individual living a gluten free lifestyle to learn the necessities of label reading as well as get some suggestions on low calorie, extremely tasty meals they can make on their gluten free diet.

The ultimate goal of this bundle is to take several problems that fitness minded individuals on a gluten free diet have and provide the solutions to those problems in one package.

In short, several problems, one solution.

Maybe you're a parent, maybe you're a business man or woman, maybe you're a college student, maybe you're none of these things. What I do know is that you live in 2016 and beyond which means your time is both limited and valuable. With that in mind I'm not going to bloat this introduction with unnecessary information just to make the bundle a little bit longer. Instead, I'm going to congratulate you. I'm going to congratulate you on taking a step, maybe the first, in understanding your gluten sensitivity or desire to be on a gluten free diet. As well as taking steps to a healthier lifestyle. Whether you're a parent, a business man or woman, college student, or none of the above, living a healthier lifestyle is never a bad idea.

Wait a minute…

What am I saying…

IT'S A GREAT IDEA!!

So stop reading this introduction and get moving to the meat of this book.

Seriously… what are you still doing here, GO!

Book 1

Gluten Free Fitness

Beginners Guide to 10 Tasty Diet Meals to Lose Weight

By Scott Jay Marshall II

©2016

What You Are Going To Learn

In this book I am going to tell you about 10 of THE BEST meals for anyone on a gluten free diet that I personally used to LOSE 60 LBS.! This is for those people out there trying to lose weight, keep calories low, or simply enjoy a healthy lifestyle. I'm not a ghost writer and I'm not a random guy picking a profitable subject to write about. I am a gluten intolerant man myself and have been living this lifestyle for years. I've done it the unhealthy way and the healthy way. Since you purchased this book, I know you've made the right decision and have decided to make healthy changes in your life. You'll learn about the foods you need to make these meals, as well as, a little bit of background on each item. Also, you'll discover how to prepare these items and how much of these items to have. Furthermore, you'll read how to serve these dishes and even visit a key factor to weight loss and a healthy lifestyle overall, calories. In general, the media, world, and people make losing weight and living a healthy lifestyle way more complicated than it should be. Especially when factoring in special dietary needs like gluten free (GF) eating. These meals are super easy to prepare with simple, 100% gluten free ingredients packed full of goodness.

Disclaimer

This book was written as a suggestive guide to creating healthy meals and losing weight with 100% gluten free foods. Before starting this or any other diet/weight loss program speak with your physician. The writer, distributors, and all others involved with this book are not responsible for any negative results that manifest from following the suggestions in this work. Please ensure you are buying high quality, healthy, and clean produce and foods to ensure you do not contract a foodborne illness. Always sanitize your food prep area before preparing these meals. Starting with high-quality ingredients in a sanitary environment is crucial, especially when preparing meats and other perishable food items. Lastly, inspect the cooking surfaces and tools you will use before use to ensure they are sanitary and functioning properly.

Table Of Contents

A Special Thank You - Free Gift

As a special thank you for purchasing my book, I would like to give you my irreplaceable guide to 5 of the most commonly overlooked foods containing gluten. These 5 foods get gluten free folks in trouble thousands of times a day, every day, all over the world. This is mostly because you would never think about them containing gluten.

So please accept my free gift, *The Hidden Gluten Report*. Make sure YOU know 5 of the most commonly overlooked glutinous foods on the market. You'll thank yourself for it and you'll be able avoid these major downfalls in your gluten free diet. Without this report you may eat them tomorrow, the next day, or maybe even today. This amazing report is FREE so don't miss out and take the risk of eating these glutinous foods. Unfortunately, it won't be free forever, so claim your copy now.

Claim Your FREE Copy

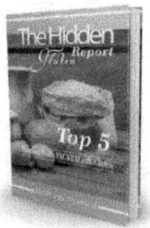

Just to give you a heads up, you'll be asked for your email address. I ask for 2 reasons:
1) So I know where to send your FREE gift.
2) You're obviously an intelligent, diet minded individual living a gluten free lifestyle or trying to help someone close to you.

With this in mind, I will periodically send out email notifications about additional free promotions, valuable gluten free information and discounts on my other gluten free books in the *Gluten Free Fitness* series. I NEVER spam and will always respect, and keep your email private.

Download Your FREE Copy Of "The Hidden Gluten Report"

Why Should You Trust What I'm Telling You?

Hey, that's a fair question, right? "Who's this guy telling me what's what about gluten?" On May 3, 2008, at approximately 11:30PM was the first time my gluten allergy surfaced. Some people say stressful situations make the allergy finally manifest, some say physical trauma. Whatever it was, that's when mine started. I didn't know what was going on at first so I continued to compound the problem over the coming months. At the time, I had a high amount of gluten in my diet—burgers, cereals, glutinous alcohol, chips, chicken strips, toast, you name it. Foods with gluten in them were my favorite kinds of food and I ate them all the time. With all of these compounding problems working against me problems came on quick and didn't go away until I changed my diet. I was constipated, had low energy levels, lost weight because my body wasn't getting the nutrition it needed and more.

My quality of life and health were not good.

Then, a friend with Celiac disease casually mentioned symptoms he experienced after eating gluten. They were too familiar to ignore at that point. We looked up a list of issues related to gluten allergies and found I had 18 out of 20 symptoms. So, I started eating gluten free or at least close to it. I was so new to this diet that I didn't know what had gluten in it except for the obvious items like bread. As any Celiac or gluten free dieter eventually learns, it's hidden in foods you would never expect to have it. I'll tell you more about that later.

Slowly, my health improved. The more disciplined I became with my diet the better I felt. I started gaining healthy weight back, constipation was no longer a problem, and I didn't feel super tired anymore.

Life started getting better and my health grew alongside it.

I didn't return fully to normal until I had completely cut gluten out of my diet, and even then it took awhile to get it out of my system.

Years later, I gained weight and finally decided to start eating better for good. Just because you eat gluten free doesn't mean you are consuming healthy food. So I researched and learned how to eat gluten free while staying healthy. Many of the health foods on the market or ingredients in supposedly healthy recipes have gluten (i.e. noodles, grains, granola bars, etc.). At first, it seemed like someone was asking me to dig the car out of the snow with a spoon—painful and tedious. However, after a lot of studying, I found it was actually quite easy to eat healthy and gluten free simultaneously.

You can't have the donuts or sugary cereals the company brings in for breakfast. And, you should avoid the five pieces of cake and cookie dough ice cream at any birthday party.

Before long, I had lost 60 pounds, was much happier, had started putting on muscle, and was looking lean.

At long last, my health and quality of life had reached what I would describe as nothing short of amazing.

I want to share what I learned with other people wanting to follow a gluten free diet. You can have AMAZING meals, keep calories low, not sacrifice taste or enjoyment, support a healthy weight loss plan, and do it 100% gluten free.

In short, that's why you should trust what I'm telling you. I've walked the walk and talked the talk when it comes to eating and being physically fit on a gluten free diet. Like any other healthy lifestyle, it takes commitment, discipline, and drive. You will find a gluten free lifestyle is far beyond worth it.

I'm going to assume since you bought this book, you have goals aligned with living a healthy lifestyle, enjoying satisfying food, losing some weight, and doing it gluten free. I'm here to tell you, I believe in you and know you can do it.   series and beyond.

What Is Gluten And What Is A Gluten Free Diet?

Gluten is a mixture of different proteins found in wheat and other related grains. Some refer to gluten as a "binding protein" because it often gives bread and other products it's chewy texture and feel. For example, take a raw piece of wheat, get it wet, and grind it between your fingers. You would find it produces a white, sticky substance—also known as gluten.

A gluten free diet consists of a meal plan comprised of items 100% void of the protein(s) known as gluten. This is sometimes difficult for many reasons:

1. Wheat is cheap and is used as a filler for many different products. It is also added as a thickening agent in some foods.

2. As a direct result of #1, gluten free items can be expensive if the food item you are buying is traditionally made with gluten. Bread and soups would be a good example of those types of items. A standard loaf of gluten free bread can cost as much as $6 or more.

3. Some food companies are tricky when it comes to labeling what is in their food. For example, if you look at a bottle of Powerade you are not going to see wheat anywhere on the label. However, if you read the ingredients list of some of the flavors you will find an item called modified food starch. This is a nonspecific starch comprised of nonspecific items. Many Celiacs report discomfort and negative reactions after they

consume modified food starch because one of the most common nonspecific food items used to make it is wheat.

4. You'd be surprised to know what foods actually contain gluten. For example, many brands of jerky contain gluten. It helps the flavor stick to and impregnate the meat better which helps with flavor while it sits on the shelf.

5. For all these reasons a celiac or someone following a gluten free diet has to become a label reader which some people find exhausting. In all honesty, it can be difficult but if you are following a gluten free diet it is something you will have to get used to.

It's easy to understand why so many people feel so lost when they discover they are a Celiac or are gluten intolerant and HAVE to go on a gluten free diet. However, once you learn the basics, and get a little experience under your belt it becomes second nature.

Quick Tip/Tool/Trick

If you're serious about losing weight, monitoring calories you eat is critical. Nothing does that better than a phone app like "LoseIt!" or "MyFitnessPal." I'm not paid by anyone to mention these apps so know that I'm only telling you this information because I believe they are valuable tools. I personally use "LoseIt!" but I have heard nothing but good things about "MyFitnessPal." Both applications essentially function the same way.

They are fast, simple, straight forward, have MASSIVE databases of foods, and will really help you keep on track and stay accountable. Even better, you can scan the barcodes of the foods you eat and they will automatically calculate the calories for you instead of having to manually search and enter foods you eat. They will even give you counts on nutrients like protein, carbs, fats, and more. The best part—THEY ARE TOTALLY FREE.

The late, great Greg Plitt (an extremely influential fitness model and motivational speaker) once said if you expend more calories than you take in, YOU WILL lose weight. CLICK HERE TO WATCH THE VIDEO. What did he mean? Let's say you are eating 2500 calories a day to maintain your current weight. If you decrease it to 2300 calories a day while maintaining the same activity levels, the pounds will come off. It's an inarguable fact that works to your benefit because it's easy to track and it's guaranteed.

So do yourself a favor, go download a calorie tracking app and make the most out of your day and these meals. Seriously go, I'll be here when you get back.

LET'S GET COOKING!

Complete Ingredient List

This is a complete list of all the ingredients you will be using to put together these meals, as well as, a small tidbit about what makes each of these foods great.

Meats & Eggs:

- Trimmed Beef Sirloin
    - Beef is a classic protein source. It gets a bad rap because it is a red meat. Truthfully, it can be extremely good for you. Especially if you trim and cook a lean cut like sirloin with healthy oils (i.e. coconut oil). What do I mean by trimming? I imply to trim off the fat. For example, in the center of a sirloin steak is a "divider," where the steak breaks in half. Trim the connecting those two pieces and any fat on the outsides of the cut as well. If you have dogs, toss the trimmings to them, they'll thank you for it.
- Trimmed Pork Sirloin
    - Like beef, pork often gets a bad rap and in many cases for good reason. It IS higher in fat than other protein sources. However, you can take steps much like those steps I mentioned with beef to ensure you are getting the leanest protein possible while still allowing variety into your healthy lifestyle. Just like the beef, choosing a cut like a sirloin is ideal. It's already the more lean cut but you can also decrease the fat by trimming and cooking in healthy oils.
- Ground Turkey Burger
    - While I have seen turkey burger come in ratios as fatty as 73/27 (73% meat, 27% fat), turkey burger is

exceptionally lean and tasty. It's one of my favorites and I have seen it as lean as 93/7. You'll want to watch it closely while cooking if you use that ratio as the lower fat ratios burn easily because of less moisture. That's where a good healthy oil comes in. If I feel like biting into a cheesy taco but don't want to overindulge and go over my calories for the day, I make a nice batch of turkey burger tacos. They are a staple around my house.

- Lean Ground Beef Burger
  - Choosing to use a lean ratio and drain the fat from the pan as you are cooking your beef burger can make it a superior high source of protein. And, let's face it, a burger is just plain delicious.
- Chicken Breasts
  - Big surprise right? Anyone who has seen a picture of a fitness meal prep or heard someone talking about eating healthy, the chicken breast was involved for good reason. Virtually no carbs or fats, and more than 5 grams of protein per ounce. BAM! If that's not a fitness yummy, I don't know what is.
- Chicken Thighs
  - Some people suggest darker chicken meats like thighs and drumsticks can be ideal for athletes. The reason? Breast tends to be much more expensive than thighs and drumsticks because it's the staple/ideal white chicken meat everyone loves. Besides cost, the fat is another reason. Right about now you're saying, "Wait back up, fats? I thought fats were bad." No, they are not. They are a necessity. While fats are broken down too slowly to be used as energy during workouts, they are an essential piece of all hormone production. In short, if you are a gal, fat helps you produce and maintain healthy estrogen levels. If you're a bro, the same goes for you but with testosterone as opposed to estrogen. Check out

THIS ARTICLE from www.livestrong.com to learn more.

- Fish
    - It's hard to make a bad choice when it comes to fish. While salmon is, of course, the fitness food of choice, fish in general are high in protein, have virtually no carbs, and are low in bad fats. THIS ARTICLE from *Men's Journal* suggests that the best fish are salmon, albacore tuna, mackerel, and trout. So, bust out the fishing pole fisherman and catch yourself a fitness dinner!
- Turkey Sausage Patties (pre-cooked)
    - Turkey sausage is not only lower in fat, and calories than pork sausage but it tastes amazing. At this point in my life, I prefer it. With the right spices, it tastes the same as pork sausage and isn't anywhere near as greasy. I hate the feeling of tasting more grease than meat at breakfast.
- Eggs
    - Eggs, as some would say, are nature's perfect food. There is a lot of debate about cholesterol, so if that concerns you, just have egg whites instead. Separating the yolk from the white is easy enough when you crack it or you can simply buy egg whites.

Fruits & Veggies:

- Russet Potatoes
    - A staple of any table, russet potatoes are cheap, hearty, and filling.
- Red Potatoes
    - Red potatoes are the bees knees of potatoes. They are naturally gluten free, fat-free, help with energy levels, blood pressure, and even stress. Not to mention they taste excellent.
- Sweet Potatoes

- Some call sweet potatoes one of the world's healthiest foods. It's packed full of vitamins and minerals, has an almost sweet taste, and is inexpensive.
- Granny Smith Apple
  - Truly the apple of the fitness world. Protein and fiber in one shot, they contain vitamins, minerals, antioxidants and even fight some digestive disorders. Plus, they're tasty.
- Kale
  - I LOVE kale. Yup, kale, the plant some people think is only for decoration. Often associated with a bitter taste, kale is often referred to as a superfood. It's hard to eat it the wrong way if you are into the green tasting foods. I prefer my kale raw, or blended in a smoothie with fruit and protein.
- Spinach
  - Another super food of the greens world. There is a reason they had the classic cartoon character Popeye munching this stuff down. Spinach is packed full of all the powerful things you would expect from a green superfood but is much milder in taste compared to kale.
- Bell Peppers
  - Bell peppers come in a multitude of colors and sizes but are all basically the same. They are not hot at all as some people would suspect with "pepper" in the name. They have a very mild flavor in fact.
- Green Beans
  - Green beans belong in any fitness meal plan. Also known as string beans, they are extremely beneficial for you and even promote bone health. Not something you'd expect from a vegetable, I know.
- Broccoli
  - Broccoli is actually a member of the cabbage family. High in fiber and protein, broccoli was one of Thomas Jefferson's favorites.

- Cauliflower
  - Cauliflower is an amazing plant both for its health benefits and alternative uses. I suggest you look up "garlic cheese bread from cauliflower." You can thank me after your taste buds chill out.
- Carrots
  - One of my personal favorites, carrots are packed with beta-carotene which our bodies turn into Vitamin A. In fact, it's one of the best sources for Vitamin A in the world which is why they are so good for our vision, bones, and teeth.
- Asparagus
  - Another personal favorite, yes, really. That weird vegetable that makes your pee smell funny. Three years after planting, asparagus reaches it's growing season and can grow as much as 6 inches PER DAY.
- Strawberries
  - Strawberries taste fantastic and are one of the best sources of antioxidants in the world.
- Blueberries
  - Full of fiber and perfect in a muffin, blueberries are excellent for you and are exceptionally tasty. They are also a strong source of antioxidants. This fruit CAN be expensive if you buy them at the wrong time of year.
- Bag of Greens
  - A mixed bag of greens will be used. This can be whatever tickles your fancy—Asian mix or power greens to name a couple.
- Banana
  - Not just for monkeys, bananas are one of the best sources of potassium around. Keep them on hand if you commonly experience charley horses in your muscles and you'll find that come less often. They are also ideal for an energy boost and sustained blood sugar levels right before a workout.

- Cucumber
  - Cucumbers taste crisp and clean, are extremely inexpensive, and are basically tubes of water with skin so they are an awesome choice to add to salads or eat in slices to help with hydration.

Other:

- Protein Powder
  - A must-have for anyone going through strenuous workouts. For approximately 45 minutes after a workout, your body is going to be screaming for protein to put the muscle fibers you just tore back together. Absorbing protein in liquid form via protein shakes allows your body to digest it faster and easier which means your body gets more out of it when it needs it most.
- Instant Oatmeal
  - Often overlooked in fitness and diets, oatmeal is full of fiber and extremely tasty when you add cinnamon or fruits. Instant oatmeal is better if you are going to use it in the morning when time is short. And, there are TONS of gluten free instant oatmeal on the market that taste excellent.
- Cinnamon
  - Cinnamon helps sustain healthy insulin levels, has anti-inflammatory properties, has been linked to heart disease prevention, is full of antioxidants, fights several types of infections, and the list goes on. Cinnamon is one those spices you should keep in your diet at all times. If you don't enjoy the flavor, it does come in capsule form.
- Yogurt
  - What type you get is totally up to you. Greek yogurt, plain, key lime, some type of fruit yogurt—it's hard to go wrong with a good yogurt. The best kinds will

come with live, active cultures for your digestive system.

- White Rice
  - White rice is inexpensive, goes with almost anything, and is extremely low in calories.
- Brown Rice
  - Brown rice shares the same benefits of white rice but is an even better grain choice for you. It's high in fiber, helps keep blood sugar levels in check, and studies show it supports the reduction of high cholesterol levels.
- Butter
  - Yes, butter in a diet book. People often assume that eating healthy means not eating foods you really enjoy. This is not the case. Instead, you practice control and don't go overboard. For example, I will use small amount of butter for one meal in this book.
- Lemon Juice
  - Lemon juice is inexpensive and adds a kick to a lot of different foods. It's available in all different kinds like organic, and all natural. This citrus juice can be found at almost any grocery store, and is virtually calorie free.
- Some Standard Seasonings
  - Salt, black pepper, garlic salt, onion powder, chopped and dried onions.

Now that we have our complete list of items, let's put them to good use.

A Quick Word On Amounts

I'm going to give amounts for each item of the meals. However, feel free to modify these amounts as you see fit to line up with your dietary needs and fitness goals. Just understand as you add more, the calories of the meal will increase. And, if you take food away, the calories will decrease.

LET'S GET TO IT!!!

Meal # 1 - Steak & Taters

Ingredients:

- 8 oz. trimmed beef sirloin
- 1 russet potato
- 1 sliced bell pepper
- Standard Seasonings (to taste)

Preparations:

- Rinse off your potato and poke holes in it with a fork for a faster cook time. Then wrap it in tin foil.
- Cut up your bell pepper by slicing off the top, then slicing it into quarters and removing the seeds. Finally, cut it into thin strips no more than a half-inch wide.
- Make sure your sirloin is defrosted and ready to cook. If you get caught in a jam and forget to defrost it, then you can either stick it in the microwave, or you can put it in a container of HOT water until it's defrosted. When it is defrosted, take a good sharp knife and trim off any visible fat. Yes, this may sacrifice a small amount of flavor but ultimately makes it a healthier meal.

Making The Meal:

1. Get your potato cooking first since it takes the longest to cook. You can cook it in a standard oven, a toaster oven, or as a last resort, the microwave. The first two options will

produce a much better result. Generally, a baked potato can take an hour to cook so squeeze in a workout or something else productive while it cooks. If you're using the microwave the amount of time will vary.

2. After your potato has been cooking for about 40-45 minutes in the oven, grab a healthy oil like coconut oil and throw it into a pan. It doesn't take much. Then season and cook your steak to your liking—rare, medium rare, medium well, well done. When you have 5 minutes left of cooking the steak, throw in the strips of bell pepper. This will blend the flavors of your steak and peppers. Cook the peppers long enough to still have their crisp snap.

3. To serve, slice your steak into strips and put them on a plate with your peppers so they can be eaten together in a single bite and place your baked potato on a small plate on the side. Feel free to add salt, pepper and a small amount of butter to your potato but stay away from cheese to keep things low in calories. Then, of course, enjoy.

Meal # 2 - Fish & Veggies

Ingredients:

- 1 fillet of your favorite type of fish
- 1 head of broccoli
- ½ head of cauliflower
- 2 carrots
- ¼ stick of butter
- Standard Seasonings (to taste)

Preparations:

- Rinse off your broccoli, cauliflower and carrots, as you always should with your produce.
- Make sure your fillet is defrosted and ready to be cooked.

Making The Meal:

1. Preheat your oven to around 450°F. Season your fish with lemon juice, garlic salt, onion powder, and pepper. Check your fish periodically. Depending on your oven, cook time should be between 35-45 minutes. To test the fish and make sure it is done, just stick it with a fork and see if it comes apart easily.
2. While your fish is cooking, melt a SMALL amount of butter in a dish to brush your over your broccoli and cauliflower. Then add a small amount of salt and pepper and begin to steam them. If you don't have a steamer, then you can either stir fry

the veggies in a pan with some healthy coconut oil or you could eat it raw. Raw is my personal favorite. You don't lose any of the nutrients through the cooking process and I find having a cold crisp food to counter the cooked meat is excellent.

3. To serve, combine all of the vegetables in a large bowl and place fish fillet on a small plate and enjoy.

Meal #3 -The Gobbler Burger Special

Ingredients:

- 10-12 ounces of ground turkey burger. You will lose a lot of the weight during the cooking process like you will with any ground meat. Cooked, you'll end up with 6-8 ounces which is an ideal amount for a single serving when you are on a fitness diet. Protein is ESSENTIAL to any fitness diet.
- 1 cup of rice
- 2 carrots
- 1 handful of asparagus
- Standard Seasonings (to taste)

Preparations:

- Make sure your turkey burger is defrosted. If you forget to defrost ahead of time, turkey burger will defrost rapidly. Simply put it in hot water for a few minutes. Only until you can easily break the turkey burger apart. It's SO much easier if you have meats separated ahead of time because it allows you to defrost and manage them easily.
- Rinse and cut the tops and bottoms off of your carrots and the bottoms off of your asparagus. I like to cut my asparagus in half horizontally but I'll leave that up to you. Next, take your carrots and cut them in half, and then cut them in half long ways. I recommend a sharp knife and SLOW, CONTROLLED movements. It's easier to cut yourself than you would think.

Making The Meal:

1. Start the rice first. If you are using 5-minute rice, then still do it first so it can be out of the way. OF COURSE, make sure while you are shopping for this white rice, you find a white rice labeled gluten free because not all white rice is gluten free.

2. Get your turkey burger cooking in a pan. This time, do not use any cooking oil. The water that is expelled from the turkey burger will be more than enough to prevent it from burning unless you are using a very lean ratio. Then a little coconut oil would be appropriate. Fair warning, turkey burger cooks much faster than beef burger so be on the lookout for that. To make sure it's done, make sure there is no amount of pink leftover in the middle or anywhere else. Poultry should always be thoroughly cooked for safety. Season with salt, onion powder, and black pepper. This isn't in the ingredient list but if you would like you can research poultry herb mixes to use as well.

3. In this recipe, the carrots and asparagus are meant to be served raw. This is one of my all time favorite lunch meals. If you would like you could steam them or throw them into the pan with your turkey burger once it has completely cooked. If you do give it a try and stay open-minded, I think you will really enjoy the combination of cooked and raw foods.

4. To serve, mix your turkey burger and rice together in a large bowl. Then place your carrots and asparagus on a small plate and dig in!

Meal # 4 - Piggy & Beans

Ingredients:

- 8 oz. of trimmed pork sirloin
- 1 cup of brown rice
- 7 oz. of green beans (approx. half of a standard can)
- Standard Seasonings (to taste)

Preparations:

- Measure 1 cup of brown rice into a bowl or cup.
- Open your can of green beans. If you're not getting it from a can then simply eyeball half of a can's worth. You can put plastic over the can and save the other half for later, or cook it all now and save the cooked portion in the fridge to be eaten later.
- Make sure your pork is defrosted. Just like I discussed with the beef sirloin, you are going to want to trim your pork sirloin. Typically, the pork sirloin will be fattier than the beef sirloin so you are going to have more to trim. Again, practice safety, and use a sharp knife to carefully do your trimming.

Making The Meal:

1. Prepare your rice in a rice cooker first. Brown rice generally takes longer to cook than white rice so follow the directions on the package you bought. Also, make sure you buy a brand specifically marked gluten free. Just like I discussed with white rice, not all brown rice brands on the market are

gluten free. So, do your research and make sure it's gluten free before you waste your money and buy it. This shouldn't be difficult. Labeling foods as gluten free has become a strong marketing point for food manufacturers and producers.

2. Put your beans in a pot with water and start cooking them on a medium heat until they are soft and break easily with a spoon or fork.

3. While your rice and beans cook, pull out a pan and melt some healthy oil like coconut oil down in the pan. Pork has a tendency to stick to the pan so make sure you cover the entire pan surface with the oil. Pork should be cooked THOROUGHLY. Season with garlic salt, onion powder, black pepper, chopped and dried onions. If you decided to research poultry herb mixes give that a shot as well. Mmm, delicious!

4. Serve everything together on a single plate and enjoy.

Meal # 5 - Author's Choice

Ingredients:

- 2-3 medium sized chicken thighs. Chicken loses a lot of it's weight during the cooking process and you want to end up with approximately 8 oz. of cooked chicken which the 2-3 thighs should provide.
- 1 cucumber
- 1 carrot
- 1 large or 2 medium sized red potato(es)
- Standard Seasonings (to taste)
- Cinnamon

Preparations:

- Rinse off the cucumber, carrot, and potatoes.
- Cut the tip and bottom off the carrot and slice it diagonally into circular slices.
- Slice your red potatoes into 8 pieces. To do this, cut it in half and then section those 2 pieces into 4. This will make it easier to cook and will help the potato absorb any seasons you choose to add.
- Slice your cucumber horizontally into circular slices about a quarter-inch thick.
- Remove the skin from your chicken thighs. To reduce cook time, remove the bone as well and slice the chicken thigh into smaller pieces. Inch wide strips should do. If you're not that confident with a knife, you don't need to remove the bone. It will just take a little longer to cook as the bone holds

a lot of cold and takes the longest to warm up, increasing cook time.

Making The Meal:

1. Take your carrot and potatoes and put them into a pot to start cooking or put them in a steamer or crock pot. They will be done when the potatoes are soft and break easily. Depending on your cooking method this will take 30-60 minutes. Do this first since it will take the longest.
2. Your cucumber is ready so no more prep needed there.
3. Throw water into a pan and get your chicken cooking at a high heat. Like pork, you want to thoroughly cook chicken until there is no pink leftover, at all. When the meat breaks apart easily and white all the way through, then you know it is done. Make sure you continue to add water during the cooking process so the meat doesn't dry out or burn in the pan. I like to use all of the standard seasonings in this recipe. I also add a small amount of cinnamon to this recipe, cinnamon is very good for you and the salty/sweet clash is amazing.
4. To serve, place your chicken, carrot slices and potatoes on a plate with your cucumber slices in a small bowl and enjoy.

Meal # 6 - The Fitness Classic

Ingredients:

- 1 large trimmed chicken breast or 2 small trimmed chicken breasts
- 1 cup of brown rice
- 1 granny smith apple
- Standard Seasonings (to taste)

Preparations:

- Measure out 1 cup of brown rice into a bowl or cup.
- For ease of eating and presentation, cut your apple into 4 sections. Remove the stem first. Next, cut your apple into quarters. Follow up by carefully slicing from top to bottom and remove the center of each slice that contains any seeds or piece of the core. Apple seeds contain cyanide and should never, ever be eaten. It would take a large amount to make you sick but it's best to just avoid them altogether.
- Make sure that your chicken breast defrosts all the way through. With a sharp knife, remove any excess fat that is on the breast.

Making The Meal:

1. Similar to meal 4, prepare your rice in a rice cooker first. Brown rice generally takes longer to cook than white rice so follow the directions on the package you bought. Again,

make sure you use gluten free brown rice marked gluten free on the package.

2. Place a small spoonful of coconut oil or any other healthy oil that you choose into a pan and make sure it covers the entire surface of the pan. Cook the chicken breast at medium to high heat until it is white all the way through and comes apart easily. I know I'm beating a dead horse here but ALWAYS cook chicken thoroughly. Season with black pepper, onion powder, garlic salt, and a small dash of cinnamon. Trust me, it's good.

3. To serve, cut the chicken breast into strips or chunks and mix it into the brown rice with your apple slices on a small plate on the side and munch away.

Meal # 7 - Patties, Greens & Skinny Sweets

Ingredients:

- 10 oz. of lean ground beef
- Half a sweet potato
- 2 cups of spinach
- Standard Seasonings (to taste)

Preparations:

- Rinse your spinach and sweet potato.
- Cut your sweet potato in half lengthwise and either put the other half away or cook both halves now and save one for later. I recommend the latter. Potatoes do not keep well after the insides have been exposed to oxygen.
- Put your defrosted ground beef into a Ziploc bag and add your desired ratios of the standard seasonings. Now seal the bag and mash everything together. This will make clean up of your pan later much easier and will ensure even seasoning distribution. You can apply this same technique to ground turkey. Next, take your ground beef and separate it into 2 balls of equal size. Then, flatten the balls into a patty. To keep your burgers from rising into a dome when you cook them, put a small dent in the middle of each patty with your knuckle or a spoon.

Making The Meal:

1. Wrap your sweet potato in tin foil and throw it in the oven at 450°F or in your toaster oven at the same temperature. Throw it in flat side down. You will know it is done when you push on the potato and it easily sinks in. This will take 45-60 minutes depending on the size of your sweet potato and oven.

2. Place your spinach in a bowl and cover it with your favorite salad dressing or leave it as is. Feel free to add other veggies if you want but I'm restricting it to spinach to stick with the recipe.

3. Put your hamburger patties into a pan and cook to your preference—well done, medium well, and so on. There is no need to add extra seasoning since you did it earlier. After flipping your burgers for the first time, remove them and set them on a plate and drain the grease from your pan into an old coffee can or another container that won't melt. Then put your patties back into the pan and finish cooking them. This will make the meal even leaner.

4. Serve with the patties and sweet potato on a plate with your spinach in a bowl on the side and enjoy.

Meal # 8 - Buff N' Stuff Breakfast

Ingredients:

- Your favorite flavor of gluten free instant oatmeal
- Cinnamon
- 1 scoop of protein powder
- ½ cup of blueberries
- 5 strawberries
- 1 cup of kale

Preparations:

- Get your blender or magic bullet out for your shake.
- Rinse your blueberries, strawberries, and kale.
- Remove the leafy part of the kale from the stem and toss the remains.
- Using a straw (you can see videos of this on YouTube) remove the center and leaves from your strawberries. Then using a sharp knife, cut them in half. If you don't have straws on hand you can just cut and remove the center or leave the center. Just make sure you at least remove the leaves and stem from the top.

Making The Meal:

1. Following the directions on the package, cook your instant oatmeal in the microwave. When it is done, add cinnamon and stir it in thoroughly for even distribution.

2. While your oatmeal cools, put your kale, blueberries, strawberries and protein powder into your blender along with a small amount of water, it doesn't take much. If you are using a smaller bullet style blender, then blend everything except the protein powder first. Add the protein powder and do one more quick run.
3. To serve, sit down at the table with a good book or view out your window. Put your shake into a large glass, enjoy your bowl of oatmeal, and fuel your morning.

Meal # 9 - Greens, Eggs & No Ham

Ingredients:

- 2 large eggs or the equivalent amount of egg white liquid if you are going that route
- 1 cup of mixed greens
- 1 cup of water
- 1.5 cups of your favorite fruit
- 2 ice cubes (if you have sensitive teeth you can leave these out or use cold fruit)
- Salt and pepper (to taste)

Preparations:

- Rinse your greens and fruit
- Place your egg whites or eggs into a bowl. Next, add salt and pepper and mix it all together with a whisk or fork.
- Pull out your blender. (A bullet is not recommended for this meal)

Making The Meal:

1. Put your eggs or whites into a pan and cook on medium heat until done.
2. Combine and blend the water, greens, fruit, and ice if you've decided to use it into your blender.
3. Serve your eggs on a small plate with your greens/fruit shake in a tall glass and enjoy.

Meal # 10 - I Woke Up Late

Ingredients:

- 2-3 prepackaged turkey sausage patties
- 1 banana
- 1 cup of yogurt (by cup I mean a single serving like you would pack in someone's lunch)

Making The Meal:

1. This meal is designed for those mornings when you have no time to make breakfast. Following the instructions, heat the turkey sausage patties in the microwave.
2. Grab your banana and yogurt while your turkey sausage patties are heating up.
3. Wrap your turkey sausage patties in a paper towel and head out the door to start your day.

A Quick Word On Meal Prepping

These ten meals are palate pleasing and good for you but sometimes you simply don't have time to cook. Well, fret not, there is a solution. To make all of this easier, spend some time on Sundays, or any free day you have, preparing your meals for the week or, at least the meal you never have time to cook. In my case, that's lunch, which is the case for many people.

All you need to do is increase the amounts in these recipes to accommodate the number of meals you want to make. If you want to have Meal #6 for lunch during a given week, cook five chicken breasts, cut up five apples, and make five cups of rice.

Invest in a good set of Tupperware and keep Ziploc bags on hand to separate the meals. For example, If I were prepping Meal 6, then I would put a breast and cup of rice in one container and my apples in another container or Ziploc bag.

The whole point behind meal prepping is to ensure you have readily available healthy meals in line with your fitness and diet goals. This is an underutilized tool in the fitness and diet world. It's easy to justify eating out when you don't have food prepared. Especially if you live a busy lifestyle. Plus, you get to have a home cooked meal rather than crap fast food or a TV dinner for sustenance.

So, do yourself a favor, utilize these meals and make larger amounts of them ahead of time. Set yourself apart from the others out there and give yourself a fighting edge in the fitness and diet game.

Conclusion

There you have it ladies and gentlemen—*10 tasty* *Gluten Free Fitness meals* to help you stay on track with your diet and weight loss goals. I sincerely hope you enjoyed the first book in the *Gluten Free Fitness* series and I want to commend you. Taking control of your health, especially on a gluten free diet, is hard and takes a lot of character and drive. So congratulations! You're one of the proud folks who have decided to live a better, healthier life. You rock!

A Favor To Ask

I must ask you for a favor. If you thought this guide was valuable, please leave me a review on Amazon (CLICK HERE). It would really help me out and would help this book reach more gluten free eaters. For those readers who don't know, reviews are one of the key factors to any Kindle book's success and ranking. Also, please share it with your other gluten free friends on Facebook, Instagram, Twitter, YouTube, Periscope, Snapchat, WHEREVER!

If sharing this book could help another gluten free eater get healthy, lose weight, and become more fit, then what are you waiting for?! Sometimes the only thing people need to make big changes in their lives is a little direction and motivation from a friend. When they see the success you're having, you'll inspire them to do the same.

DON'T FORGET YOUR FREE GIFT!

Again, A Special Thank You

As I come to a close, I would like to say "Thank you!" again. All of you gluten free readers and eaters are why I wrote this book and I thank you for that.

Do yourself a favor and download "The Hidden Gluten Report" ABSOLUTELY FREE!

Click Here & Claim Your FREE Copy

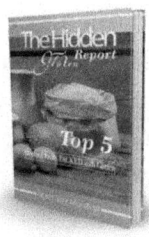

You'll learn about the 5 most commonly overlooked glutinous foods on the market. I may sound like a broken record at this point but I spent YEARS eating these without knowing I was eating gluten. It was only through extensive research, and some very uncomfortable days that I learned the truth. DON'T WAIT! It won't be free forever.

Download Your FREE Copy Of "The Hidden Gluten Report"

I Dedicate This Book…

…to the many health and fitness idols I have had over the years. My father, the late Greg Plitt, Bruce Lee, author and personal trainer Dale L. Roberts, and so many others.

As always, a dedication must go to my wonderful wife who is the foundation and core of my strength, heart, and essence. You are, and always will be, the best fan I have or will ever. I love you sweetheart.

About The Author

Scott lives amongst the purple, snow capped mountains in Northern Utah. He has lived amongst the red sand of Southern Utah as well. He lives there with his wife and 2 German Shepherds. He grew up in the area and has always had a passion for fitness. Scott is the creator of the "Doing It Better" YouTube Channel/vlog, is an avid social media buff, and loves sharing content. He loves writing about a variety of subjects including but not limited to fitness, dogs, self help, and more. He enjoys sharing stories and ideas with entrepreneurs around the world and believes that there are few people in this world that don't have something to teach, share, create, and be.

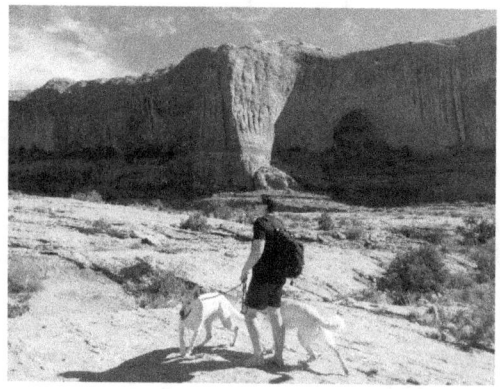

Gluten Free Fitness - Beginners Guide to 10 Tasty Diet Meals to Lose Weight

By Scott Jay Marshall II

©2016

Book 2

GLUTEN FREE FITNESS

The Ultimate Guide to Becoming a Label Reading Master

By Scott Jay Marshall II

©2016

Disclaimer

This book was written as a simple guide to reading the labels of food products to identify glutenous ingredients. This does not replace any medical advice received from a medical professional nor is this book providing any medical advice. If you ever have a severe reaction to a food item you have consumed, immediately schedule an appointment with your doctor to address the issue. The writer, distributors, and all others involved with this book are not responsible for any negative results that manifest from following the suggestions in this work. Always practice the utmost diligence when eating new foods if you have a food allergy.

After all, the few extra seconds it will take to read a label is a lot easier, cheaper, and comes with a lot less suffering than guessing.

Table Of Contents

A Special Thank You - Free Gift

As a special thank you for purchasing my book, I would like to give you my irreplaceable guide to 5 of the most commonly overlooked foods containing gluten. These 5 foods get gluten free folks in trouble thousands of times a day, every day, all over the world. This is mostly because you would never think about them containing gluten.

So please accept my free gift, *The Hidden Gluten Report*. Make sure YOU know 5 of the most commonly overlooked glutinous foods on the market. You'll thank yourself for it and you'll be able to avoid these major downfalls in your gluten free diet. Without this report, you may eat them tomorrow, the next day, or maybe even today. This amazing report is FREE so don't miss out and take the risk of eating these glutinous foods.

Claim Your FREE Copy
Or visit scott332.wix.com/hiddenglutenreport

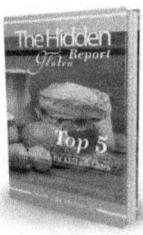

Just to give you a heads up, you'll be asked for your email address. I ask for 2 reasons:

1) So I know where to send your FREE gift.
2) 2) You're obviously an intelligent, diet minded individual living a gluten free lifestyle or trying to help someone close to you. With this in mind, I will periodically send out email notifications about additional free promotions, valuable gluten free information, and discounts on my other gluten free books in the *Gluten Free Fitness* series. I NEVER spam and will always respect, and keep your email private.

Download Your FREE Copy Of "The Hidden Gluten Report"

Introduction

It's happened to every gluten free eater out there. You were POSITIVE that it was gluten free when you ate it but you still ended up dealing with the side effects of the gluten. Were you really sure though? Did you make sure that what you were about to eat was gluten free before eating it? I'll be honest and transparent, every time I "got glutened" it was because of an oversight on my part. I made an assumption I shouldn't have made, to avoid an awkward conversation I took someone's word that something was gluten free and many others. Ironically, the biggest culprit was also the ultimate solution to the problem, I didn't read the label.

Label reading is the only way to be 100% positive that something is gluten free. You can take friend's words for it and make assumptions and get away with it for a long time but eventually, it's going to catch up with you. Life has a funny way of deciding when it wants to catch up with you. Maybe you're at a wedding, out with a group of friends, on a first date? All 3 are very good examples of times when it would be bad to "get glutened". You need to be sure.

In this book, I am going to teach you how to become a label reading master. All the way from the simple and obvious things to look for to the complicated stuff that makes you say "Really? I have to look for that?" I'm going to tell all. It's taken years of living a gluten free lifestyle and more than a gut ache or two to figure these things out. Not only figure them out but be able to communicate it in this short guide without overloading you with information. I would have paid a hundred over what you paid for this book in the beginning of my journey to avoid all the long nights and bad days "getting glutened" has caused me. So are you ready to become a master?

Let's get to it.

Claim Your FREE Copy
Or visit scott332.wix.com/hiddenglutenreport

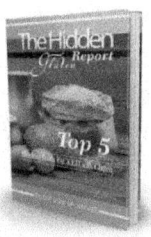

What do I mean when I say "Become a Label Reading Master in 24 Hours!"?

I read a lot of books (mostly audio) and too often I see people trying to make unnecessarily lengthy books just for the sake of having a long book because they think no one is going to take their book seriously unless it's a billion pages long.

I don't agree with this approach.

We live in a society now that like no other time in history demands action from us every second of the day. Fitting in listening to an audiobook while you drive to the grocery store. Sending an important email while your kids eat dinner. Whatever the case may be, few of us have the time to sit down, grab a book and proceed to read through 500 pages to figure out how to do something or understand something. We simply don't have that kind of time anymore. The world is evolving around us every day and the way we take in information needs to evolve as well. It needs to be more direct, to the point and provide the most value and impact.

I want to bring you the information that you need in as little time as possible without leaving out unnecessary information. I can serve you better this way and provide you with more value.

So back to the question of "What do I mean when I say "Become a Label Reading Master in 24 Hours!"? ". I mean that you can easily take in the information in this book and be able to actively apply it within 24 hours. Whether you listen to it, read it in a digital format on your phone or kindle device, or on a physical copy you can get through it in one day and be on your way back to your busy schedule with a new weapon in your gluten free arsenal.

Maybe you're an executive, maybe you're an assistant, a teacher, a doctor, a mother, a father, a student, an athlete, or any number of things. No matter what, you're a human being and your time is valuable and I respect that.

So let's get this information downloaded into that brain of yours and get you back to doing what you do.

Who Am I To Talk To You About Label Reading?

You know, I'd be asking the same thing if I was reading this book. "Who is this guy trying to tell me how I should be reading the labels of the foods I eat?" "What gives him the right?" Exceptionally valid question you have there, let me tell you why.

In May of 2008, my gluten intolerance surfaced. I remember it down to the day and time. (May 3rd, 2008 at approximately 11:30PM). It was like being stabbed with a knife in my stomach. Now, granted, this is not the most common side effect of a surfacing gluten allergy but for me, it signified a major change in my life that would impact me in ways I didn't know at the time.

In the beginning months, I had no idea what was going on. I was getting skinnier all the time, felt tired and sluggish on a constant basis, and never felt like I was getting any energy after I was eating.

Not to mention bloating, constipation and more. Sorry...I hope you weren't eating just now.

Bottom line, life was not great.

Eventually, I figured out what was going on with the help of a friend that also had a gluten allergy. In many ways, my world got turned upside down. I was the poster child for picky eaters at the time. Nothing but meat and potatoes for me. "Vegetables, fruits, what are those?" That was my general theory when it came to my diet. Chicken nuggets and strips, corn dogs, bread, you name it. If it had gluten in it, it was probably a main staple in my diet and I loved it.

As you can imagine this made grocery shopping time an exceedingly annoying pain in the butt. On top of having a food allergy, I was picky. For a long time, I cheated. Eating gluten free foods when I knew I shouldn't because I just couldn't resist but that caught up to me. I didn't feel better until I started reading labels and paying attention to what I was eating.

After a while, my lack of energy and bad eating habits started to take it's toll on my body. I started gaining weight in a big, and extremely unhealthy rate. (Not that there is a healthy rate to get to being obese.) At one point I weighed more than 100 pounds more than I did in high school. I hit 228 pounds and realized things had gotten out of control. I was unhappy, not healthy by any stretch of the imagination, I hated looking at myself in the mirror and didn't have energy for anything.

Thank goodness for a healthy diet, exercise, and label reading. Thanks to paying attention to my diet, exercising and reading labels I was able to drop 60 pounds, get healthy, improve my attitude towards life, become a professionally published author, and improve all the relationships in my life.

At this point, you're probably saying "Whoa Scott, back the train up. How did label reading, time at the gym and a healthy diet accomplish any of that." Again, that's a valid question you have. It's really quite simple. When we eat a diet that doesn't agree with us, we feel like crap. Period. When you feel like crap it bleeds into all the other aspects of your life.

Think about it.

Picture the last time you accidentally had gluten and remember how awful you felt. Did you feel like spending time with your significant other, spouse, or children? Did you feel like exercising or reading a great book? No, you felt like sitting there and waiting for the awful feeling to go away.

That is the power of becoming a label reading master. With a few simple tricks up your sleeve and some powerful knowledge, you can avoid that crappy feeling and all the negative ripples it spreads into the rest of your life. You can feel great on a consistent basis, and know that you have total control over what is going into your body. Because YOU are a label reading master, and YOU won't be caught off guard.

So master in training, shall we begin?

Claim Your FREE Copy
Or visit scott332.wix.com/hiddenglutenreport

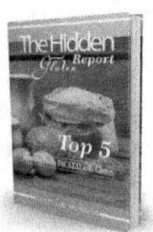

Why is all this label reading stuff necessary?

Getting "glutened" sucks, it just does. You eat something and it tasted amazing and all of the sudden you're sicker than a dog. This is a dumb problem to have and for the most part, short of a few exceptions is extremely easy to avoid.

It ALL comes down to reading labels.

Reading labels is the only way to be sure that you're not about to be "glutened". Is it irritating, yes? Does it take time, yes? Are you going to feel sorry for yourself because not everyone else needs to do that, yes? However, it's a lot easier than being sick.

The difficulties I just listed are mostly only present in the beginning. Eventually, you will come to a point where it makes you feel like you are in control of what you're eating and you will enjoy it. Eventually, it becomes second nature.
Think Daniel-san in the karate kid. At first the whole "wax on - wax off" thing was annoying and irritating and required some thought. Fast forward to the end of the movie and his habits are in place. He no longer had to make the conscious effort to do it, it was second nature.

So to answer the question "Why is all this label reading stuff necessary?", I say it's necessary because you deserve to eat good food and not worry about it afterwards. It's necessary because your health depends on it. It's necessary because you're worth it.

An Unfortunate Reality

 Unfortunately, I have to share a sad reality with you. In this day and age, food manufacturing companies are continuing to look for sneaky, back door, devious ways to avoid labeling the fact that their products contain gluten. How cheap gluten can be and it's availability make it far too appealing for many companies to steer clear of. Fitness products are in no way whatsoever an exception to this rule. If you're looking at a pre-workout, protein powders and more it's rare to find versions that are gluten free. That's not to say they aren't out there, but they are difficult to find without taking the time to look.

Because of this I have to be transparent with you and tell you that no matter what measures you take, no matter how diligent you are, no matter how much I share with you, there will be an ever-present possibility of being "glutened". The idea is to avoid it as much as you can with simple measures. To be honest, as a gluten intolerant individual and someone that has been "glutened" on several occasions, I am thankful I don't have a life-threatening allergy to something like peanuts or shellfish.

At the end of the day be thankful for the health you have. Be thankful that you have a plethora of information out there to help you avoid gluten and that you have the financial and technology means to access it. Also, be thankful you don't have to deal with an allergy that requires you to take an EpiPen everywhere in order to feel safe.

Claim Your FREE Copy
Or visit scott332.wix.com/hiddenglutenreport

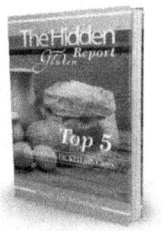

What To Look For

At the end of this book, I will share an image that will show you a mind-boggling list of things that could potentially contain gluten just so that I am thorough. However, I have found over my many years of experience that there are a few main things to watch out for. Avoid these, and you will be good to go 99% of the time.

In this section, I will go over these major offenders. I will tell you how to identify and avoid them. With a little discipline and learning, you'll be a master in no time.

The "Allergy Information" Section

This one is pretty obvious but I would feel like I've slighted you if I wasn't thorough. On most food items with a label out there, you will find an "Allergy Information" section on the back with the rest of the nutritional info. As celiacs and/or gluten intolerant individuals we are looking out for "Contains: Wheat". If there are other allergens in this section, it doesn't matter. (Unless of course you have other food allergies.) Some would have you believe that because wheat is the last item there isn't enough to bother you. This is a dangerous line of thought. Any gluten is too much gluten.

Checking the allergy information section should be your very first step. Once you've cleared the allergy information section and it doesn't contain wheat, you can move on to the more difficult to identify stuff.

Modified Food Starch

Let me be clear about this one. In this specific example, I am talking about "Modified Food Starch". Not "Modified Corn Starch", not "Modified Potato Starch", but "Modified Food Starch".

In a letter sent to one Ms. Marie Kawaguchi, founder of the Celiac Association of Northern Utah, the FDA states the following in regard to "Modified Food Starch".

"...the starch process used in preparing modified food starch removes the protein (i.e., gluten) component. Thus, modified food starch is the common or usual name of the
product regardless of source. Although we acknowledge the possibility that traces of protein
might occasionally trigger an adverse reaction, and we acknowledge your concerns, we have not
been able to document reported cases of food intolerance to the modified food starches
commonly available for commercial use. Thus, irrespective of the source, modified food starch
is not likely to be a problem for most gluten intolerant consumers. Therefore, in the absence of

information showing that modified food starch will trigger adverse reactions, there is no basis at
this time to require source declaration." You can find the article HERE. If you are reading this on paperback, please go to this address: http://bit.ly/1Y9JJ8c

That's what they say. However, I don't particularly buy it.

Whether things have drastically changed since then or they are flat out lying I just don't believe it. Keeping in mind that I am only gluten intolerant (NCGI - non-celiac gluten intolerant) and not specifically a celiac, I have on more than one occasion consumed some type of food item and ended up with negative side effects only to find that the item contained modified food starch. In my personal opinion seeing "Modified Food Starch" on the food's nutritional label is as much of a "no - go" as seeing "Contains: Wheat". It's simply not worth the risk.

I share these pieces of mastery level advice because they have served me well, not because I read them online somewhere. Every time I consume food with "Modified Food Starch", without exception, I experience negative side effects on one level or another. To catch this one, you are going to need to look at the actual ingredients list. It could be at the beginning, it could be at the end, or it could be in the middle. It doesn't matter. Yes, the order of foods in the ingredients list dictates the percentage of that item found in that particular food but like I say said before, "Any gluten is too much gluten."

So to conclude this particular section, I say this. Just don't.

The FDA says one thing but my body says another so go with your gut, best judgment, and experience here. If you asked me if you should or not, I'd tell you that you were CRAZY if you said you were going to try it. As they say, JMHO. (Just my honest opinion.) Although I'd like to make a slight alteration. JMHMO (Just my honest master's opinion.)

May Contain Traces Of Wheat

For celiacs, this is not a gray area in any way what...so...ever. Some NCGI folks say that this is a gray area for them. I disagree. I'm not saying that they are liars I'm just saying that "Any gluten is too much gluten." If you have a problem with gluten, you have a problem with gluten. Period. Remember how I talked about "Modified Food Starch" being as bad as "Contains Wheat"? This isn't any different. You may get lucky every now and again with this one but eventually, you are going to get screwed and glutened and it's going to suck. Do yourself a favor, check the allergy sections, and don't screw yourself over.

All that you are looking for is a section underneath the standard allergy section. It will clearly state "May contain traces of..." This list will often contain items like tree nuts, peanuts, and wheat. Unless you have other allergies, I assume you know what to be looking for.

Wheat, it's wheat.

Foods Without A Label

This one is trickier to handle because there isn't a label for us to flat out read and check. Being a health and/or fitness minded individual you will run into this problem mostly when buying bulk foods. What do I mean by that? Let's examine it.

Let's say you are at a health foods store and you are going to go buy bulk rice out of the big bins that health food stores always have. You will most likely find a plethora of different kinds of rice but not all rice is created equal. Some are glutinous, some are not. If you're lucky you'll be at a health food store that specifically labels the bins as gluten free or not but you may not be that lucky. In this situation, you'll have to do some detective work.

Bust out the trusty smartphone or research on your computer at home ahead of time and confirm whether or not the type of rice you are about to buy is glutinous or not. You don't want to drop a bunch of money on a bunch of food you can't eat especially when you keep in mind that most places don't accept returns of bulk foods like rice because of safety concerns.

When it comes to other label-free foods like fruits, vegetables, and unprocessed meats, you are generally safe. Note that I said "unprocessed" meats. Many of your typical deli slice style lunch meats will be glutinous. It's a super bummer but it's true. I only say "generally" because there may be some super uncommon fruit or vegetable that contains gluten but if there is I've never heard of it. Making fruits and vegetables a part of your gluten free diet is critical as we miss out on a lot of vitamins and minerals by steering clear of glutinous foods.

In conclusion, eat lots of fruit, eat lots of vegetables, and when it comes to unlabeled bulk foods make sure you are doing your detective work before you spend your hard earned money.

Sauces & Condiments

This one catches people off guard all the time. Let's say you're at a family barbecue and someone cooked up steak, chicken, or something else like that. You may initially think to yourself "Awesome, it's just meat so I'm good to go."

STOP!

No, it's really not good to go. The meat portion is, of course, good to go but stop and think about the sauce. Here's the real deal. Too often condiments and sauce companies secretly and or openly use wheat as a thickening agent. Bottom line, they use less actual product but by mixing in wheat the main product (flavoring, etc...)

goes further. Less initial expensive product and more end result product equals more profit.

Sad to say but if you can't get a look at the bottle of condiment/sauce that they used on (x) then you can't eat it. Luckily, if you eat at family's homes very often they will quickly pick up on this and either save the bottle or actively look for gluten for you. Trust me, this doesn't happen overnight but with good family, it WILL eventually happen. I'm lucky enough to have an amazing family like my parents Scott and Dixie and my in-laws Mark and Natalie that are always looking out for me.

If you're not lucky enough to be in comfortable enough situations like that then you are going to have to start to be okay with saying "No thank you, I can't eat that but I appreciate it.". Like I mentioned earlier some people have a hard time with this but it's really not that big of a deal. If someone is offended enough by you saying no to their dinner item because of an allergy then they are the one with issues, not you.

Lunch Meats

Yup, I said lunch meats.

I know, major bummer, right? Well, that's just the unfortunate reality of it. A lot of processed lunch meat manufacturers these days are using gluten as a filler item. Why they think it's a good idea to add wheat to meat is a good idea I'll never know but it's happening right now none the less. You need to keep an eye out for that hopefully ever present "Gluten Free" symbol or flat out words.

Like I talked about in the last section, don't automatically assume you are good to go just because it is meat. Stay safe and check your labels people.

Gluten Free Symbols:

Right now in business, our society, and marketing, having a gluten free product is something that people are advertising. Why are they doing this, because more and more people are getting diagnosed with celiac disease and gluten intolerance. Not to mention those that are hopping on the gluten free train because of dieting choices. Some are bodybuilders, some are athletes, some have health problems where inflammation can be an issue, the list goes on. The one thing that all these people have in common is that they create a market for gluten free products. So if I am the manufacturer of a gluten free product you better bet your butt that I'm going to advertise it.

How are they going to do this, I'll tell you. They are going to say "Gluten Free" on the label like I talked about earlier or they are going to use a gluten free symbol. I'd show you what "it" looks like but there are so many it would be impossible. What I can do is send you somewhere that will show you the mass majority of the possible symbols you are going to see.

If you are viewing this on a kindle or digital device, go to THIS LINK. If you are viewing this in a paperback copy of the book visit http://bit.ly/1sXWJEt

The Massive List

As promised, I want to share this image I came across with you. I am unsure of the original source of the image so I can't share that but I wanted to convey how serious label reading is. All of these items have the potential to contain gluten. However, like I said before the items I discussed earlier in this section are the major offenders and what you should be looking for on a regular basis to stay safe

Ingredients to Avoid in a Gluten Free Diet

Abyssinian Hard (Wheat triticum durum)
Atta Flour
Barley Grass (can contain seeds)
Barley Hordeum vulgare
Barley Malt
Beer (most contain barley or wheat)
Bleached Flour
Bran
Bread Flour
Brewer's Yeast
Brown Flour
Bulgur (Bulgar Wheat/Nuts)
Bulgur Wheat
Cereal Binding
Chilton
Club Wheat (Triticum aestivum subspecies compactum)
Common Wheat (Triticum aestivum)
Cookie Crumbs
Cookie Dough
Cookie Dough Pieces
Couscous
Criped Rice
Dinkle (Spelt)
Disodium Wheatgermamido Peg-2 Sulfosuccinate
Durum wheat (Triticum durum)
Edible Coatings
Edible Films
Edible Starch
Einkorn (Triticum monococcum)
Emmer (Triticum dicoccon)
Enriched Bleached Flour
Enriched Bleached Wheat Flour
Enriched Flour
Farina
Farina Graham
Farro
Filler
Flour (normally this is wheat)
Fu (dried wheat gluten)
Germ
Graham Flour
Granary Flour
Groats (barley, wheat)
Hard Wheat

Heeng
Hing
Hordeum Vulgare Extract
Hydroxypropyltrimonium Hydrolyzed Wheat Protein
Kamut (Pasta wheat)
Kecap Manis (Soy Sauce)
Ketjap Manis (Soy Sauce)
Kluski Pasta
Maida (Indian wheat flour)
Malt
Malted Barley Flour
Malted Milk
Malt Extract
Malt Syrup
Malt Flavoring
Malt Vinegar
Macha Wheat (Triticum aestivum)
Matza
Matzah
Matzo
Matzo Semolina
Meripro 711
Mir
Nishasta
Oriental Wheat (Triticum turanicum)
Orzo Pasta
Pasta
Pearl Barley
Persian Wheat (Triticum carthlicum)
Perungayam
Poulard Wheat (Triticum turgidum)
Polish Wheat (Triticum polonicum)
Rice Malt (if barley or Koji are used)
Roux
Rusk
Rye
Seitan
Semolina
Semolina Triticum
Shot Wheat (Triticum aestivum)
Spelt (Triticum spelta)
Spirits/Alcohols

Sprouted Wheat or Barley
Stearyldimoniumhydroxypropyl Hydrolyzed Wheat Protein
Strong Flour
Suet in Packets
Tabbouleh
Tabouli
Teriyaki Sauce
Timopheevi Wheat (Triticum timopheevii)
Triticale X triticosecale
Triticum Vulgare (Wheat) Flour Lipids
Triticum Vulgare (Wheat) Germ Extract
Triticum Vulgare (Wheat) Germ Oil
Udon (wheat noodles)
Unbleached Flour
Vavilovi Wheat (Triticum aestivum)
Vital Wheat Gluten
Wheat, Abyssinian Hard triticum durum
Wheat amino acids
Wheat Bran Extract
Wheat, Bulgur
Wheat Durum Triticum
Wheat Germ Extract
Wheat Germ Glycerides
Wheat Germ Oil
Wheat Germamidopropyldimonium Hydroxypropyl Hydrolyzed Wheat Protein
Wheat Grass (can contain seeds)
Wheat Nuts
Wheat Protein
Wheat Triticum aestivum
Wheat Triticum Monococcum
Wheat (Triticum Vulgare) Bran Extract
Whole-Meal Flour
Wild Einkorn (Triticum boeoticum)
Wild Emmer (Triticum dicoccoides)

As you can see the list is quite extensive but again I listed the major culprits above because they are what you need to look out for the majority of the time.

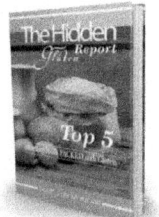

Habits Of A Master

It's easy to see now how just trusting that food is gluten free simply isn't safe, effective, or the right way to do it. You need to be absolutely sure something is gluten free before you eat it.

Just to really drive this point home, here is the definition of absolute: "complete and total"

To become a master you are going to have to set up certain habits. It takes weeks to fully develop new habits so make sure you stick with it. After all, if you are gluten intolerant or have celiac disease this is something you are going to be dealing with for the rest of your life so you better set up master level habits now or pay apprentice level habit consequences. Let's go over each one of these steps and determine what you'll need to do to accomplish them and implement them effectively in your everyday life.

Question Everything

As soon as you have decided to eat something you should be asking yourself, "Do I know this is gluten free?" Asking this question may seem obvious and a big "No duh." but it's really not.

I can't tell you how many times I asked this question on something I would never have expected to contain gluten and it actually did. To find out the top 5 hidden sources of gluten, check out the free gift at the beginning, ending, and chapter endings of this book. When all is said and done, if you haven't asked yourself this question and the answer wasn't yes, you shouldn't eat what you're about to eat. Period. There really isn't any wiggle room here.

Never guess, know.

Read The Label Every Time

Another "No duh." but again it's not. It's the whole premise of this book. As you walk through the grocery store, gas station, Wal-Mart, wherever and decide you are going to buy something, turn that thing around! It's not hard. If you're reading or found this audiobook then you OBVIOUSLY have the ability to read and look out for the items I discussed earlier in the book. No one ever said that dealing with a food allergy would be easy but these are the things that a master does. They do what is necessary to get the job done and they make sure it's done the right way. So do your due diligence, read the label, and don't get glutened!

Read the label. Every single time.

When There Isn't A Label You Need To Do 1 Of 2 Things

If it's a fruit or vegetable then you are nearly guaranteed to be okay. If however it is something like a piece of meat at a family bbq with bbq sauce on it or chips and dip at a picnic, then it's a little more complicated.

1. You can either flat out ask if you can see the label for the food which at a family member's or friend's event shouldn't be a big deal.

2. If you're uncomfortable asking then you can simply ask what kind of sauce, dip, chips that they used and look it up yourself on the web. I find that the second option is often the easiest. It's so common for people to be on their phones these days that no one is going to think twice about you hopping on the net right after you ask.

What To Do When You Are Eating Out

This is always a tricky one. There are however a few habits you can set up to help you navigate the beast of eating out when you are eating gluten free. Not only can these tips help keep gluten away from you, it will also help support your fitness goals.

Do Your Research Ahead of Time

The best and the hopefully obvious thing you could/should be doing if you have the opportunity is to research places before you go there. Do they have gluten free options? What are other people with gluten issues saying about this place? Do they have an online list of gluten free foods? These are the things you should be researching. If you can find out what you can/want to eat before going it makes ordering a lot faster and easier.

Just Ask

Simply ask if the restaurant has a lot of any experience dealing with gluten free people. Not unlike what I discussed earlier about people being aggressive with labeling their gluten free products because it is a large marketing point, restaurants are also proud of their ability to accommodate gluten free folks. It lets them stand out in the marketplace and establishes a whole new customer base. So in short, if they know what they're doing with gluten free people, they'll happily say yes to your question.

Communicating From The Start

Let's assume that you couldn't do ahead of time research because it was a spur of the moment outing to the restaurant. Let's also assume that you've asked if the restaurant commonly accommodates gluten free patrons. Now it's time to state the fact that you have a gluten allergy. Some places will have no idea of what to do and some will already know exactly what they are doing. Either way, you've now done your part and established that you do in fact have a food allergy which I think we can agree is an important factor.

Cross Contamination

This is your opportunity to ask about how they handle their gluten free patrons. A lot of the time you'll go somewhere that has gluten free options like substituting leaf lettuce for a bun on a burger to make it gluten free but they cook your beef on the same grill top that they just toasted buns on for example. You'll need to ask if they take special precautions to make sure that cross-contamination does not take place. Places like Red Lobster have an excellent setup to handle gluten free patrons. They have a whole process from using cleaned/different cooking surfaces, uncontaminated utensils and more. Plus they have a killer steak, I recommend the New York.

Gluten Free Options

Now is when you will want to ask if they have a gluten free menu. If they don't have a gluten free menu some places will have gluten free indicators throughout their menu. Some will indicate that a food is gluten free. Some indicate that alterations can be made to the dish to make it gluten free. Like I brought up earlier, some places will allow you to make simple changes like switching out a burger bun for leaf lettuce. This is one of those times that your gluten allergy is supporting your fitness goals. You're not getting the excessive carbs or calories from the bun. Some buns depending on if they are buttered, have onions, and so on can contain as many as 400-500 calories. THAT'S CRAZY! Not only that but you'll be getting a little more green into your diet. (Even though lettuce is mostly water.) If you really want to go that extra mile in regards to your fitness goals, ask if they have kale leaves, that'll really make it a fitness burger for champions. Bottom line, ask what their gluten free options are so you can make the best decision possible for your fitness goals and your allergy.

Sauces, Glazes, and Dressings

One of the times that people get themselves into trouble is with toppings. Sauces, glazes used on meats while they were cooked, dressings for salads, and other condiments like ketchup and mustard can contain gluten so you need to be careful here. Unless you're getting a bbq burger then it's unlikely that your burger has any type of glaze or ahead of time sauces that were applied to it so you are fairly safe there. However, if you were to order something like say, shredded roast beef or sliced ham, then you need to ask questions. "Was the glaze on the ham / beef used during the cooking process gluten free?" "Was glaze of any kind used at all?" Don't be surprised if your server has to ask the kitchen about this one. The others are up to you. If you are adding bbq sauce to your burger or steak, if you're adding ketchup and mustard to your burger, if you're adding dressing to your salad, you're going to need to READ THE LABEL before you put it on your food.

Beware Of The French Fry

You may be thinking to yourself "Ummm, fries are potatoes which are gluten free so I'm good to go." Well, you're mostly / half right. A plain ole' potato cut into french fries would be totally fine. (As long as you're not having too many, gotta watch those calories.) The problem comes when they are "special" fries. No, not pot french fries but fries that come with extras. A lot of the time you will come across places that have french fries that are battered. You can recognize this by looking at the fry. Generally, you'll see a normal french fry with what looks like crusties all over it. This happens a lot with curly fries like you would find at Arby's. What you need to do is ask ahead of time when you are ordering and ask if they are battered. If they are not battered then you are good to go. If you forget to ask before you order and you get a plate of the fries with "crusties", it's best to just leave them alone. You can ask for a replacement item like a baked potato or salad but you shouldn't eat those "crusty" fries.

Eating out when you are trying to maintain a fitness diet and a gluten free lifestyle can be a bit tricky but these habits are what allow me to hit my calories every day and totally avoid gluten even though I'm eating out with friends and family. Make these habits yours and you can enjoy the same health and social freedom.

Habits Of A Master Wrap Up

Look, I know it's irritating. I know it's about zero fun and I know that it's especially hard if you are new to a gluten free diet. Not to mention that you are already watching your calories and/or macros to get those #glutenfreefitnessmaster gains...or losses, HA! As you can tell, I love to let my personality jump off the page and don't stick to the standard "writing rules".

In all seriousness, this stuff can be a major pain in the ass when you are having to deal with a food allergy on top of the struggles and challenges of living a fit lifestyle. Weigh-ins, calorie counting, macro tracking, exercise routines, the list goes on. They all take their toll and adding these habits to the mix doesn't make it any easier. However, there is a silver lining. You'd be surprised at what you would find if you were to google all the bodybuilding/fitness benefits of a gluten free diet. YES! There are crazy people out there doing this to themselves on purpose, but for good reason. Do some research and I think you'll be surprised.

Claim Your FREE Copy
Or visit scott332.wix.com/hiddenglutenreport

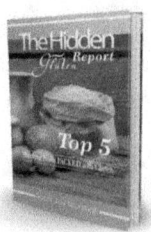

Master's Review: What Was Covered

1. An Unfortunate Reality

   a. Unless you are some type of magician the numbers say you are going to "get glutened at some point. The tools and habits I've shared with you will give you a HUGE advantage in avoiding that for as long as possible.

2. Who Am I To Talk To You About Label Reading?

   a. I've been living a gluten free lifestyle for 8 years now, I have MORE than put in my 10,000 hours. I share this advice with you because it reliably works for me day by day, every day.

3. Why All Of This Label Reading Stuff Is Actually Necessary.

   a. This is all necessary because you can't go through your life assuming if you have a gluten intolerance problem. You just count. Regardless of your friend's good intentions, or how much you THINK what you're about to eat is gluten free, you have to be sure. The only way to do that is to read the label.

4. What Items To Look For On Your Food Labels.

    a.   I went over EXACTLY what you need to be looking for. I told you about the ways people are trying to trick you, and I even shared an OVERWHELMING list of possible culprits. Most importantly I showed you the major offenders and how to avoid them.

5. What To Do When You Don't Have A Label On Your Food.

    a.   Sometimes life isn't what we would call ideal. It would be great if everything had to list every allergen it contained but that's not the case. So, I went over some tips and tricks to surface the unlabeled world, the family bbq, or even the night out with your friends or sweetheart.

6. The Habits You Need To Implement and Stick To Obtain Label Reading Master Status.

    a.   No one becomes a master overnight, you'll need to put in your time as an apprentice. That being said, with some time and effort you can gain mastery. You can turn your chaos of "is this gluten free?" into a habit of knowing whether it is or isn't. No more guessing, only knowing.

7. Free Gift ([CLICK HERE](#))

    a. For anyone wanting to take their Gluten Free Fitness lifestyle to the next level. (Go to this address if you are reading this on paperback: scott332.wix.com/hiddenglutenreport.)

Keeping all of these things in mind is essential. You can't simply implement some but not all of what I discussed in this book, it just doesn't work that way. You can't put oil in a car, a nice set of tires, give it a full tank of gas, but no spark plugs and expect it to run. All the pieces of the puzzle are necessary. You MUST read labels, you MUST implement strong habits, you MUST be sure about foods before eating them, you MUST use your access to the internet to confirm foods without labels or that you didn't prepare are safe to eat. You must do all of these things every day, all the time, no exceptions. Hey, no one ever said becoming a Gluten Free Fitness Label Reading Master would be easy, but for people like us, it is necessary. You can either take these tools I have placed in your hands and use them like a master to keep yourself safe and healthy, or you can constantly run the risk of being glutened. Which, we all know really, really, really sucks.

Claim Your FREE Copy
Or visit scott332.wix.com/hiddenglutenreport

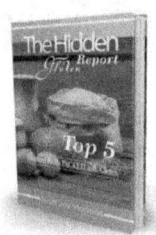

Conclusion

Lots to take in I know. However, with all this information at your disposal, I have no doubt that in no time at all you will become a label reading master. In the end, it all comes down to one thing, the mindset of a master.

A master does not do what is easy, nor does he or she take the easy way out. They identify their needs, and they exercise character and discipline to get it done. That is what you are, you are a master in training that is going to do what it takes to become a full-fledged label reading master.
You can use these principles to simply ensure all gluten has been cut from your life, or you can become a Gluten Free Fitness master and truly take a hold over your fitness world and health.

You have an issue with gluten, that's not something you can't change. What you can do is come to a realization, a realization that is the motivating force behind my publishing. Helping people come to the realization that regardless of your gluten issue, it is not a limitation, it is simply an obstacle. One that is easily overcome with a little master training and discipline. So, in conclusion, I leave you with this:

"Stop looking at your gluten issues as a limitation. Kick your constant fear of accidentally eating gluten to the curb, become a gluten free fitness master, and take control of your life and your health."

    -Scott Jay Marshall II
    Husband
    Gluten Free Fitness Master
    Author/Publisher
    Doggy Daddy

A Special Thank You - Free Gift

As a special thank you for purchasing my book, I would like to give you my irreplaceable guide to 5 of the most commonly overlooked foods containing gluten. These 5 foods get gluten free folks in trouble thousands of times a day, every day, all over the world. This is mostly because you would never think about them containing gluten.

So please accept my free gift, *The Hidden Gluten Report*. Make sure YOU know 5 of the most commonly overlooked glutinous foods on the market. You'll thank yourself for it and you'll be able to avoid these major downfalls in your gluten free diet. Without this report, you may eat them tomorrow, the next day, or maybe even today. This amazing report is FREE so don't miss out and take the risk of eating these glutinous foods.

Claim Your FREE Copy
Or visit scott332.wix.com/hiddenglutenreport

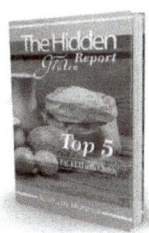

Just to give you a heads up, you'll be asked for your email address. I ask for 2 reasons:

3) So I know where to send your FREE gift.
4) 2) You're obviously an intelligent, diet minded individual living a gluten free lifestyle or trying to help someone close to you. With this in mind, I will periodically send out email notifications about additional free promotions, valuable gluten free information, and discounts on my other gluten free books in the *Gluten Free Fitness* series. I NEVER spam and will always respect, and keep your email private.

Download Your FREE Copy Of "The Hidden Gluten Report"

About The Author

Scott lives amongst the purple, snow capped mountains

in Northern Utah. He has lived amongst the red sand of Southern Utah as well. He lives there with his wife and 2 German Shepherds. He grew up in the area and has always had a passion for fitness. Scott is the creator of the "Doing It

Better" YouTube Channel/vlog, is an avid social media buff, lives a gluten free lifestyle and loves sharing content. He loves writing about a variety of subjects including but not limited to fitness, dogs, self help, and more. He enjoys sharing stories and ideas with entrepreneurs around the world and believes that there are few people in this world that don't have something to teach, share, create, and be.

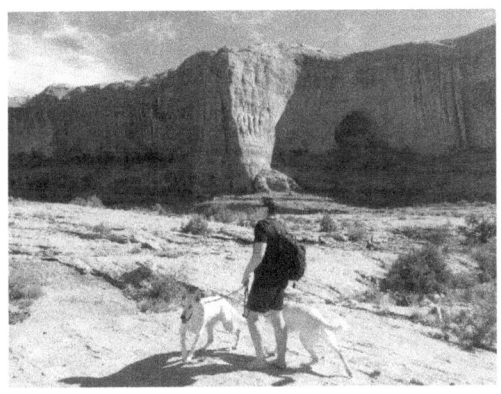

Other Publications

Gluten Free Fitness: Beginners Guide to 10 Tasty Diet Meals to Lose Weight
Click Here or visit http://amzn.to/1YdsbrH

Connect With Me

- Instagram: #glutenfreefitnessmaster
- YouTube: http://bit.ly/GFFitMasterYouTube
- Facebook: http://bit.ly/GFFitMasterFacebook
- Twitter: @GFFitMaster
- SnapChat: GFFitMaster
- Beme: gffitmaster

www.ingramcontent.com/pod-product-compliance
Lightning Source LLC
Chambersburg PA
CBHW060638290526
45793CB00001B/307